VAGUS NERVE REVIVAL

A Practical Manual For Minimizing Anxiety And Depression + Strategies For Alleviating Stress And Enhancing Emotional Resilience

DR. KYREN STEVEN

Copyright © 2024 By Dr. Kyren Steven

All Rights Reserved...

Table of Contents

Introductory 6

CHAPTER ONE 10

   Importance Of Vagus Nerve Function 10

   Definition And Significance Of Vagal Tone 15

CHAPTER TWO 20

   Factors Affecting Vagal Tone 20

   How Vagal Tone Impacts Health . 24

   Vagus Nerve And Its Role In The Mind-Body Connection 30

CHAPTER THREE 36

   Stress Response And The Vagus Nerve 36

   Techniques To Improve Mind-Body Harmony 41

CHAPTER FOUR 47

Physical And Mental Health Benefits Of Vagus Nerve Stimulation 47

Deep Breathing Techniques........53

Diaphragmatic Breathing Exercises 60

CHAPTER FIVE 67

Box Breathing And Its Benefits ...67

Yoga Poses And Sequences That Stimulate The Vagus Nerve 73

Yoga's Impact On Vagal Tone 80

CHAPTER SIX 87

Mindfulness Practices And Their Effects On The Vagus Nerve........87

Aerobic Exercises And Their Impact On Vagal Tone............................95

CHAPTER SEVEN 102

Resistance Training And Vagus Nerve Stimulation 102

Nutrients And Foods That Support Vagus Nerve Function...............109

CHAPTER EIGHT...........................117

Cold Exposure And Vagal Response 117

Massage Therapy And Its Effects On The Vagus Nerve 123

CHAPTER NINE 131

Creating A Daily Routine...........131

Conclusion.................................138

THE END 140

Introductory

The vagus nerve, also known as the tenth cranial nerve or CN X, is one of the longest and most complex nerves in the body. It is a mixed nerve, meaning it contains both sensory and motor fibers, and it is responsible for a wide range of functions related to parasympathetic control of the heart, lungs, and digestive tract.

Here are some key functions and features of the vagus nerve:

• **Parasympathetic Control**: The vagus nerve plays a major role in the parasympathetic nervous system, which is responsible for rest and digest functions.

It helps regulate heart rate, breathing, and digestive processes such as peristalsis (contractions that move food through the digestive tract) and the secretion of digestive enzymes.

- **Sensory Functions**: It carries sensory information from the throat, larynx (voice box), heart, lungs, and most of the abdominal organs back to the brain. This sensory feedback helps regulate autonomic functions and provides information about the state of the body to the brain.

- **Motor Functions**: The vagus nerve also has motor functions, controlling muscles in the throat (involved in speech and swallowing) and in the digestive tract. It helps regulate the production of stomach acid and the contraction of stomach muscles.

- **Role in the Brain-Gut Axis**: It is crucial in the communication between the brain and the gut, known as the brain-gut axis. The vagus nerve carries signals from the gut to the brain that can influence mood, stress levels, and even immune responses.

- **Other Functions**: Beyond its primary roles in autonomic functions and gut-brain communication, the vagus nerve has been studied for its potential role in treating conditions such as epilepsy and depression through methods like vagus nerve stimulation.

Overall, the vagus nerve is essential for maintaining homeostasis in the body, regulating numerous physiological processes, and facilitating communication between the brain and various organs.

CHAPTER ONE
Importance Of Vagus Nerve Function

The vagus nerve plays a crucial role in several important functions within the body, highlighting its significance in overall health and well-being:

• **Regulation of Heart Rate**: The vagus nerve is a key component of the parasympathetic nervous system, which helps regulate heart rate and maintain cardiovascular homeostasis. By influencing the sinoatrial node of the heart, the vagus nerve helps slow down the heart rate when necessary, contributing to overall heart health.

• **Respiratory Control**: It provides motor innervation to the muscles involved in respiration, particularly the diaphragm and the muscles of the larynx. This enables precise control over breathing patterns and ensures efficient gas exchange in the lungs.

- **Digestive Processes**: The vagus nerve is heavily involved in the regulation of digestion. It stimulates the production of stomach acid and enzymes, enhances gastrointestinal motility (movement of food through the digestive tract), and facilitates nutrient absorption. Dysfunction of the vagus nerve can lead to digestive issues such as gastroparesis (delayed stomach emptying).

- **Brain-Gut Communication**: Through its sensory fibers, the vagus nerve plays a critical role in the bidirectional communication between the brain and the gut, known as the brain-gut axis. This communication pathway influences mood, stress responses, and immune function. Proper vagus nerve function is associated with better emotional regulation and resilience to stress.

- **Inflammatory Response**: The vagus nerve has anti-inflammatory effects through its regulation of the cholinergic anti-inflammatory pathway. Stimulation of the vagus nerve can suppress excessive inflammation, which is implicated in various chronic diseases such as arthritis, inflammatory bowel disease, and even neurodegenerative disorders.

- **Role in Mental Health**: Vagus nerve stimulation (VNS) has shown therapeutic potential in treating certain psychiatric disorders, including depression and anxiety. By modulating neurotransmitter release and brain activity, VNS can improve mood and emotional well-being.

- **Seizure Control**: In epilepsy management, VNS has been used as an adjunct therapy to reduce the frequency and severity of seizures in individuals who do not respond well to medications.

The vagus nerve is integral to maintaining physiological balance and health across multiple systems in the body. Its functions extend from regulating heart rate and digestion to influencing mood and immune responses. Understanding and supporting vagus nerve function can have profound implications for overall health and quality of life.

Definition And Significance Of Vagal Tone

Vagal tone refers to the activity level of the vagus nerve, particularly its parasympathetic nerve fibers that regulate the autonomic nervous system. It reflects the balance between the sympathetic (fight-or-flight) and parasympathetic (rest-and-digest) branches of the autonomic nervous system, with higher vagal tone indicating stronger parasympathetic activity.

Significance of Vagal Tone:

- **Stress Response Regulation**: High vagal tone is associated with better stress resilience and quicker recovery from stressful events. The vagus nerve helps dampen the body's stress response by slowing heart rate and lowering blood pressure after a stressful situation.

- **Heart Health**: Vagal tone influences heart rate variability (HRV), which is a measure of the variation in time intervals between heartbeats. Higher HRV, often indicative of higher vagal tone, is associated with better cardiovascular health, including reduced risk of heart disease and improved overall heart function.

- **Digestive Health**: Strong vagal tone supports optimal digestive function by enhancing the production of digestive enzymes and promoting efficient nutrient absorption. It also helps regulate stomach acidity and intestinal motility, reducing the likelihood of gastrointestinal disorders like irritable bowel syndrome (IBS).

- **Inflammation Control**: The vagus nerve plays a role in regulating inflammation through the cholinergic anti-inflammatory pathway. Higher vagal tone can help mitigate excessive inflammation, which is implicated in various chronic diseases.

- **Mental and Emotional Well-being**: Vagal tone is linked to emotional regulation and mental health. Individuals with higher vagal tone tend to exhibit better mood regulation, reduced anxiety, and lower incidence of mood disorders such as depression.

- **Social Engagement**: Vagal tone influences social behavior and interpersonal relationships. It has been associated with better social skills, empathy, and the ability to form and maintain positive social connections.

Measurement of Vagal Tone:

- Vagal tone is typically assessed through measures such as heart rate variability (HRV), respiratory sinus arrhythmia (RSA), and responses to standardized tests of parasympathetic function. These measures provide insights into the balance and strength of the autonomic nervous system, offering valuable information for assessing overall health and well-being.

Vagal tone is a critical indicator of autonomic nervous system function, influencing cardiovascular health, stress resilience, digestion, inflammation control, and emotional regulation. Enhancing vagal tone through various practices such as deep breathing exercises, mindfulness techniques, physical activity, and social engagement can contribute to improved overall health and quality of life.

CHAPTER TWO
Factors Affecting Vagal Tone

Vagal tone, the measure of the activity level of the vagus nerve's parasympathetic fibers, can be influenced by a variety of factors. These factors can either enhance or diminish vagal tone, affecting overall health and well-being. Here are some key factors that influence vagal tone:

• **Stress Levels**: Chronic stress can lower vagal tone by activating the sympathetic nervous system (fight-or-flight response) more frequently and suppressing parasympathetic activity. Practices such as mindfulness, relaxation techniques, and stress management can help maintain or increase vagal tone.

• **Physical Activity**: Regular physical exercise, particularly aerobic exercise, has been shown to increase vagal tone. Exercise stimulates the vagus nerve, promoting parasympathetic activity and improving heart rate variability (HRV), which is a marker of vagal tone.

- **Breathing Techniques**: Deep breathing exercises, such as diaphragmatic breathing or paced breathing, stimulate the vagus nerve and can enhance vagal tone. Slow, deep breaths increase the activation of the parasympathetic nervous system, promoting relaxation and reducing stress.

- **Sleep Quality**: Adequate and quality sleep is essential for maintaining healthy autonomic function, including vagal tone. Poor sleep patterns and sleep disorders can disrupt autonomic balance and decrease vagal tone.

- **Meditation and Mindfulness**: Practices that promote mindfulness, such as meditation and yoga, have been found to increase vagal tone. These practices encourage relaxation and stimulate parasympathetic activity.

- **Nutrition and Gut Health**: The gut-brain axis involves communication between the gut and the brain via the vagus nerve. A healthy diet that supports gut microbiome diversity and reduces inflammation can positively influence vagal tone.

- **Social Connections**: Positive social interactions and emotional support can enhance vagal tone. Strong social connections and relationships are associated with better autonomic nervous system function.

- **Age and Genetics**: Vagal tone tends to decrease with age, but lifestyle factors can mitigate this decline. Genetic factors also play a role in determining individual differences in vagal tone.

- **Vagus Nerve Stimulation**: Direct stimulation of the vagus nerve, through medical devices or techniques like transcutaneous vagus nerve stimulation (tVNS), can be used therapeutically to enhance vagal tone and treat certain medical conditions.

Understanding these factors and incorporating lifestyle habits that support vagal tone can contribute to better overall health, stress resilience, emotional well-being, and cardiovascular function.

How Vagal Tone Impacts Health

Vagal tone, which reflects the activity level of the vagus nerve's parasympathetic fibers, plays a significant role in various aspects of health and well-being. Here are some key ways in which vagal tone impacts health:

• **Cardiovascular Health**: Higher vagal tone is associated with better cardiovascular function. The vagus nerve helps regulate heart rate variability (HRV), which is an indicator of how well the heart can respond to stress and adapt to changing demands. Optimal vagal tone promotes a healthy balance between sympathetic (fight-or-flight) and parasympathetic (rest-and-digest) nervous system activity, leading to better overall heart health and reduced risk of cardiovascular diseases.

• **Stress Resilience**: Vagal tone influences the body's response to stress. A higher vagal tone promotes quicker recovery from stressors by facilitating relaxation responses (parasympathetic activation), which counteracts the physiological effects of stress (sympathetic activation). Individuals with higher vagal tone tend to exhibit better stress resilience, lower levels of anxiety, and improved emotional regulation.

• **Digestive Health**: The vagus nerve plays a crucial role in digestion by stimulating the production of digestive enzymes, promoting stomach acid secretion, and regulating gastrointestinal motility. Optimal vagal tone supports efficient digestion and nutrient absorption, while low vagal tone can contribute to digestive disorders such as gastroparesis (delayed stomach emptying) and irritable bowel syndrome (IBS).

- **Inflammation Regulation**: Vagal tone influences the body's inflammatory response through the cholinergic anti-inflammatory pathway. Activation of the vagus nerve can reduce inflammation by inhibiting the production of pro-inflammatory cytokines. This anti-inflammatory effect is beneficial in managing conditions associated with chronic inflammation, such as autoimmune diseases and metabolic disorders.

- **Mental and Emotional Well-being**: Vagal tone is linked to emotional regulation and mental health. Higher vagal tone is associated with reduced symptoms of depression and anxiety, improved mood stability, and greater resilience to psychological stressors. Techniques that increase vagal tone, such as mindfulness practices and deep breathing exercises, are often used as complementary therapies in mental health treatment.

• **Immune Function**: The vagus nerve plays a role in modulating immune responses. Optimal vagal tone supports immune system balance and function, contributing to effective immune responses against infections and reducing the risk of chronic inflammatory conditions.

• **Social Engagement and Relationships**: Vagal tone influences social behaviors and interactions. Individuals with higher vagal tone tend to have better social skills, empathy, and the ability to form and maintain positive relationships. Strong social connections, in turn, contribute to better overall health and well-being.

Vagal tone impacts multiple facets of health, including cardiovascular function, stress resilience, digestive health, inflammation regulation, mental well-being, immune function, and social interactions. Enhancing vagal tone through lifestyle modifications and therapeutic interventions can promote better overall health outcomes and quality of life.

Vagus Nerve And Its Role In The Mind-Body Connection

The vagus nerve plays a pivotal role in the mind-body connection, serving as a crucial link between the brain and various organs throughout the body. Here are several key aspects of how the vagus nerve influences the mind-body connection:

• **Bi-directional Communication**: The vagus nerve facilitates bidirectional communication between the brain and the body's organs, especially the gut (gut-brain axis). This communication pathway allows the brain to influence gastrointestinal function and vice versa. For example, emotional states can impact digestive processes through vagal signaling.

• **Emotional Regulation**: The vagus nerve is involved in regulating emotional responses and facilitating emotional resilience. Higher vagal tone is associated with better emotional regulation, reduced anxiety, and improved stress management. Vagal activation can promote a calming effect on the body by stimulating parasympathetic activity, which counters the physiological effects of stress (sympathetic activation).

• **Mood and Mental Health**: Vagal tone influences mood stability and mental health. Low vagal tone has been linked to conditions such as depression, anxiety disorders, and post-traumatic stress disorder (PTSD). Conversely, techniques that increase vagal tone, such as deep breathing exercises and mindfulness practices, are often used therapeutically to improve mood and alleviate symptoms of mental health disorders.

• **Stress Response Modulation**: The vagus nerve plays a key role in modulating the body's response to stress. It helps regulate the autonomic nervous system by balancing sympathetic (fight-or-flight) and parasympathetic (rest-and-digest) activity. Optimal vagal tone supports resilience to stressors, promoting quicker recovery and reducing the negative impact of chronic stress on physical and mental health.

- **Influence on Inflammation and Immunity**: Through its anti-inflammatory effects via the cholinergic anti-inflammatory pathway, the vagus nerve can influence immune responses and inflammation levels throughout the body. Effective vagal regulation may contribute to better immune function and reduced risk of inflammatory conditions.

- **Social Behavior and Relationships**: Vagal tone is associated with social behaviors and interpersonal relationships. Individuals with higher vagal tone tend to exhibit better social skills, empathy, and the ability to form positive social connections. This aspect of vagal function underscores its role in social engagement and emotional bonding.

• **Therapeutic Applications**: Vagus nerve stimulation (VNS) is a therapeutic approach that involves direct electrical stimulation of the vagus nerve.

It has been used to treat conditions such as epilepsy, depression, and chronic pain by modulating brain activity and neurotransmitter release. VNS highlights the potential of the vagus nerve in influencing both physical and mental health outcomes.

The vagus nerve serves as a vital mediator in the mind-body connection, integrating physiological processes with emotional and cognitive states. Its role extends beyond regulating bodily functions to impacting emotional resilience, stress responses, mental health, immune function, and social interactions, illustrating its profound influence on overall well-being.

CHAPTER THREE
Stress Response And The Vagus Nerve

The vagus nerve plays a crucial role in modulating the body's stress response through its influence on the autonomic nervous system (ANS). Here's how the vagus nerve interacts with the stress response:

• **Autonomic Nervous System Regulation**: The autonomic nervous system (ANS) is divided into two branches: the sympathetic nervous system (SNS) and the parasympathetic nervous system (PNS). The SNS is responsible for the "fight-or-flight" response, activating during stress to prepare the body for action. The PNS, predominantly through the vagus nerve, counters this response by promoting relaxation and calming effects (rest-and-digest response).

• **Vagal Tone and Stress Resilience**: Vagal tone, which reflects the activity level of the vagus nerve, influences how the body responds to stress. Higher vagal tone is associated with stronger parasympathetic activity and quicker recovery from stressful events. This helps in regulating heart rate variability (HRV) and maintaining physiological balance, reducing the negative impact of stress on the body.

• **Role in Emotional Regulation**: The vagus nerve facilitates emotional regulation by connecting the brain to the heart and gut. Through its sensory fibers, the vagus nerve provides feedback to the brain about the body's physiological state, influencing emotional responses. Optimal vagal function promotes better emotional resilience and adaptive coping mechanisms in response to stressors.

• **Influence on Inflammation**: Stress can trigger inflammation in the body, contributing to various chronic diseases. The vagus nerve helps regulate inflammation through the cholinergic anti-inflammatory pathway. Vagal activation inhibits the release of pro-inflammatory cytokines, thus mitigating the inflammatory response triggered by stress.

- **Impact on Digestive Function**: During stress, blood flow is redirected away from the digestive system (to support the muscles and brain) as part of the fight-or-flight response. Vagal tone influences digestive processes by promoting optimal stomach acid secretion, enhancing digestion, and reducing symptoms of gastrointestinal disorders exacerbated by stress.

- **Mind-Body Connection**: The vagus nerve plays a critical role in the bidirectional communication between the brain and the body. It integrates emotional and cognitive responses with physiological functions, helping to maintain homeostasis and overall well-being during stressful situations.

- **Clinical Applications**: Vagus nerve stimulation (VNS) is used clinically to treat conditions associated with dysregulated stress responses, such as epilepsy, depression, anxiety disorders, and chronic pain. By modulating vagal activity, VNS can help restore autonomic balance and improve resilience to stress.

The vagus nerve acts as a key regulator in the body's response to stress, promoting adaptive responses and mitigating the negative effects of chronic stress on physical and mental health. Enhancing vagal tone through practices like deep breathing, mindfulness, and physical exercise can support stress resilience and overall well-being.

Techniques To Improve Mind-Body Harmony

Improving mind-body harmony involves practices that integrate mental, emotional, and physical well-being, fostering a balanced and cohesive relationship between the mind and body. Here are several techniques that can help enhance mind-body harmony:

• **Mindfulness Meditation**: Mindfulness meditation involves paying attention to the present moment without judgment. It cultivates awareness of thoughts, emotions, and bodily sensations, promoting a deeper connection between the mind and body. Regular practice can reduce stress, enhance emotional regulation, and improve overall well-being.

• **Yoga**: Yoga combines physical postures (asanas), breath control (pranayama), and meditation to integrate the mind and body. It promotes flexibility, strength, and relaxation while enhancing mindfulness and reducing stress. Different styles of yoga, such as Hatha, Vinyasa, or Kundalini, offer varied approaches to achieving mind-body harmony.

• **Deep Breathing Exercises**: Deep breathing techniques, such as diaphragmatic breathing or belly breathing, activate the parasympathetic nervous system through the vagus nerve. This promotes relaxation, reduces stress hormones like cortisol, and improves oxygenation of tissues, fostering a calm mind-body state.

• **Progressive Muscle Relaxation (PMR)**: PMR involves tensing and then relaxing different muscle groups systematically. This technique helps release physical tension, reduce stress, and increase body awareness. It can be practiced regularly to promote relaxation and improve overall physical and mental well-being.

- **Tai Chi and Qigong**: These ancient Chinese practices combine slow, deliberate movements with deep breathing and meditation. Tai Chi and Qigong enhance balance, flexibility, and mindfulness while reducing stress and promoting relaxation. They integrate physical movements with mental focus, promoting harmony between the mind and body.

- **Biofeedback**: Biofeedback techniques provide real-time information about physiological processes such as heart rate variability, muscle tension, or skin temperature. By learning to control these responses through relaxation techniques, individuals can enhance mind-body awareness and improve stress management skills.

- **Nature Connection**: Spending time in nature, such as hiking, gardening, or simply being outdoors, can promote relaxation, reduce stress, and enhance overall well-being.

Nature connection fosters a sense of grounding and perspective, facilitating mind-body harmony through natural environments.

- **Creative Expression**: Engaging in creative activities such as art, music, dance, or writing allows for self-expression and emotional release. Creative expression can promote mindfulness, reduce stress, and foster a deeper connection between thoughts, emotions, and physical sensations.

- **Healthy Lifestyle Choices**: Adopting a balanced diet, getting regular exercise, prioritizing adequate sleep, and managing stress through practices like time management and social support can support mind-body harmony. These lifestyle choices optimize physical health while nurturing emotional and mental well-being.

- **Mindful Eating**: Practicing mindful eating involves paying attention to the sensory experience of eating, including taste, texture, and smell. It encourages awareness of hunger and satiety cues, promoting a healthier relationship with food and fostering mind-body connection through nourishment.

By incorporating these techniques into daily life, individuals can cultivate greater awareness, resilience to stress, and overall harmony between the mind and body. Each practice offers unique benefits that contribute to holistic well-being and improved quality of life.

CHAPTER FOUR
Physical And Mental Health Benefits Of Vagus Nerve Stimulation

Vagus nerve stimulation (VNS) is a therapeutic technique that involves delivering electrical impulses to the vagus nerve, typically through a device implanted under the skin in the chest area. Here are some of the physical and mental health benefits associated with vagus nerve stimulation:

Physical Health Benefits:

• **Epilepsy Management**: VNS is FDA-approved for treating epilepsy, particularly for reducing the frequency and severity of seizures in patients who do not respond well to medications. It works by altering the electrical activity in the brain that can trigger seizures.

• **Treatment of Depression**: VNS is used as a treatment option for individuals with treatment-resistant depression (TRD). The stimulation of the vagus nerve is thought to influence neurotransmitter levels in the brain, such as serotonin and norepinephrine, which are involved in mood regulation.

• **Chronic Pain Relief**: VNS has shown promise in managing chronic pain conditions, including migraines and neuropathic pain. It may modulate pain pathways and reduce pain perception through its effects on brain regions involved in pain processing.

- **Improved Heart Health**: VNS has been studied for its potential cardiovascular benefits. It can help regulate heart rate variability (HRV), which is an indicator of cardiovascular health. By enhancing vagal tone, VNS may improve heart rate control and reduce the risk of arrhythmias.

- **Inflammatory Disorders**: VNS has anti-inflammatory effects through the cholinergic anti-inflammatory pathway. It can reduce levels of pro-inflammatory cytokines and modulate immune responses, potentially benefiting conditions associated with chronic inflammation, such as rheumatoid arthritis and inflammatory bowel disease.

Mental Health Benefits:

• **Reduction in Depression and Anxiety Symptoms**: Beyond its use in TRD, VNS has been studied for its antidepressant and anxiolytic effects. It can improve mood stability, reduce symptoms of anxiety, and enhance overall emotional well-being.

• **Enhanced Emotional Regulation**: VNS may improve emotional regulation by modulating brain regions involved in emotion processing and stress response. This can lead to better stress resilience and adaptive coping mechanisms.

• **Cognitive Function**: Some research suggests that VNS may have cognitive benefits, such as improved memory and executive function. These effects are thought to be related to enhanced neurotransmitter activity and neuroplasticity in the brain.

- **Quality of Life**: By alleviating symptoms of chronic conditions like epilepsy, depression, and chronic pain, VNS can significantly improve overall quality of life. It may enhance daily functioning and reduce the burden of symptoms on mental and physical well-being.

Considerations:

- **Individual Responses**: The effectiveness of VNS can vary among individuals, and it may take time to observe significant benefits. Close monitoring and adjustments by healthcare providers are necessary to optimize outcomes.

- **Safety**: VNS is generally considered safe, but like any medical procedure, it carries potential risks and side effects. These can include hoarseness, coughing, throat pain, and in rare cases, more serious complications related to device implantation or stimulation.

Vagus nerve stimulation offers a multifaceted approach to improving both physical and mental health outcomes. It has demonstrated efficacy in managing epilepsy, treatment-resistant depression, chronic pain, and potentially other inflammatory and neurological conditions. Ongoing research continues to explore its therapeutic potential and expand its applications in clinical settings.

Deep Breathing Techniques

Deep breathing techniques, also known as diaphragmatic or abdominal breathing, are effective practices for promoting relaxation, reducing stress, and improving overall well-being. Here are several common deep breathing techniques:

Diaphragmatic Breathing:

- **Technique**: Sit or lie down comfortably. Place one hand on your chest and the other on your abdomen. Inhale deeply through your nose, allowing your abdomen to expand while keeping your chest relatively still. Exhale slowly through your mouth, feeling your abdomen contract.

- **Benefits**: Diaphragmatic breathing helps to engage the diaphragm fully, promoting efficient oxygen exchange in the lungs. It activates the parasympathetic nervous system, inducing relaxation and reducing the physiological effects of stress.

4-7-8 Breathing (Relaxing Breath):

- **Technique**: Sit or lie down comfortably. Inhale quietly through your nose for a count of 4 seconds. Hold your breath for 7 seconds. Exhale completely through your mouth, making a whooshing sound, for 8 seconds. Repeat the cycle.

- **Benefits**: This technique helps regulate breathing and increase oxygen intake. It can induce a calming effect on the body and mind, promoting relaxation and reducing anxiety.

Box Breathing (Square Breathing):

• **Technique**: Sit upright with a straight back. Inhale deeply through your nose for a count of 4 seconds, allowing your abdomen to expand. Hold your breath for 4 seconds. Exhale slowly and completely through your mouth for 4 seconds. Hold your breath for 4 seconds before inhaling again. Repeat the cycle.

• **Benefits**: Box breathing helps to regulate the breath and balance the autonomic nervous system. It enhances focus, reduces stress, and promotes mental clarity and relaxation.

Alternate Nostril Breathing (Nadi Shodhana):

• **Technique**: Sit comfortably with your spine straight. Use your right thumb to close your right nostril. Inhale deeply through your left nostril. Close your left nostril with your right ring finger, and exhale slowly through your right nostril. Inhale through your right nostril, close it, and exhale through your left nostril. Repeat this cycle, alternating nostrils.

• **Benefits**: Nadi Shodhana balances the flow of energy (prana) in the body and calms the mind. It improves focus, enhances respiratory function, and reduces stress and anxiety.

Resonant or Coherent Breathing:

• **Technique**: Find a comfortable breathing rate (typically around 5-6 breaths per minute). Inhale and exhale deeply and evenly, focusing on a smooth and steady rhythm. Use a paced breathing app or metronome to maintain consistency.

• **Benefits**: Resonant breathing synchronizes heart rate variability with breathing rhythm, promoting coherence in the autonomic nervous system. It enhances relaxation, reduces anxiety, and improves emotional regulation.

Tips for Practicing Deep Breathing Techniques:

• **Consistency**: Practice deep breathing techniques regularly to reap their benefits. Aim for at least a few minutes of practice each day, gradually increasing the duration as you become more comfortable.

• **Environment**: Choose a quiet and comfortable environment for deep breathing exercises to minimize distractions and enhance relaxation.

• **Posture**: Maintain good posture during deep breathing exercises to optimize lung capacity and diaphragmatic movement.

• **Mindfulness**: Focus on the sensation of the breath entering and leaving your body. Stay present and attentive to the rhythm and quality of your breathing.

Deep breathing techniques are accessible tools that can be integrated into daily life to manage stress, improve relaxation, and promote overall well-being.

Diaphragmatic Breathing Exercises

Diaphragmatic breathing, also known as abdominal or deep breathing, is a technique that emphasizes the use of the diaphragm, a large dome-shaped muscle located at the base of the lungs, to achieve efficient and relaxed breathing. Here's how to practice diaphragmatic breathing exercises:

Steps for Diaphragmatic Breathing:

Find a Comfortable Position:

- Sit or lie down in a comfortable position. You can place a pillow under your knees if lying down to support your lower back.

Relax Your Body:

- Close your eyes if it helps you relax. Release tension in your muscles, particularly your shoulders and neck.

Place Your Hands:

- Place one hand on your chest and the other on your abdomen, just below your rib cage. This allows you to feel the movement of your diaphragm and helps you ensure you're breathing deeply into your abdomen.

Inhale Deeply Through Your Nose:

- Slowly inhale through your nose, allowing your abdomen to expand fully. Focus on pushing your abdomen out against your hand while keeping your chest relatively still. This movement indicates that you are using your diaphragm effectively.

Exhale Slowly Through Your Mouth:

- Exhale slowly and gently through your mouth, allowing your abdomen to fall inward naturally. You can lightly contract your abdominal muscles to help expel the air completely.

Repeat the Breathing Cycle:

- Continue this deep breathing pattern, inhaling deeply through your nose and exhaling slowly through your mouth. Aim for a smooth, relaxed rhythm without forcing your breath.

Practice Regularly:

- Start with a few minutes of diaphragmatic breathing exercises each day and gradually increase the duration as you become more comfortable. Incorporate this practice into your daily routine to experience its benefits over time.

Benefits of Diaphragmatic Breathing:

- **Stress Reduction**: Diaphragmatic breathing activates the parasympathetic nervous system, promoting relaxation and reducing the physiological effects of stress, such as elevated heart rate and blood pressure.

- **Improved Oxygenation**: By using the diaphragm effectively, diaphragmatic breathing enhances the exchange of oxygen and carbon dioxide in the lungs, improving overall respiratory efficiency.

- **Enhanced Relaxation**: This technique induces a calming effect on the body and mind, helping to alleviate anxiety, tension, and muscle tightness.

- **Support for Respiratory Health**: Diaphragmatic breathing can be beneficial for individuals with respiratory conditions such as asthma or chronic obstructive pulmonary disease (COPD), as it encourages deeper and more efficient breathing.

- **Promotion of Mind-Body Awareness**: Practicing diaphragmatic breathing increases mindfulness and body awareness, fostering a deeper connection between mental and physical well-being.

Tips for Effective Diaphragmatic Breathing:

- **Consistency**: Practice diaphragmatic breathing regularly to develop proficiency and maximize its benefits.

- **Environment**: Choose a quiet and comfortable environment for your practice to minimize distractions and enhance relaxation.

- **Posture**: Maintain good posture during diaphragmatic breathing exercises to optimize diaphragm movement and lung capacity.

- **Progression**: Gradually increase the duration of each breathing session as you become more accustomed to diaphragmatic breathing. Start with 5-10 minutes and work your way up to longer sessions.

Diaphragmatic breathing is a simple yet powerful technique that can be integrated into daily life to promote relaxation, reduce stress, and support overall well-being.

CHAPTER FIVE
Box Breathing And Its Benefits

Box breathing, also known as square breathing, is a relaxation technique that involves breathing in a structured pattern to promote calmness, reduce stress, and enhance focus. Here's how box breathing works and its benefits:

Box Breathing Technique:

Steps for Box Breathing:

• **Find a Quiet Space**: Sit comfortably with your spine straight, or lie down in a relaxed position.

• **Inhale**: Inhale deeply through your nose while counting to four. Feel your abdomen expand as you fill your lungs with air.

- **Hold**: Once you've inhaled fully, hold your breath for a count of four. Keep your lungs filled without straining.

- **Exhale**: Slowly exhale through your mouth for a count of four. Empty your lungs completely.

- **Hold**: After exhaling, hold your breath again for a count of four before beginning the cycle again.

- **Repeat the Cycle**: Continue the box breathing pattern for several minutes, focusing on the rhythm and depth of your breaths. You can adjust the duration of each count (e.g., 5 seconds instead of 4) to suit your comfort level.

- **Practice Regularly**: Aim to practice box breathing daily or during times of stress to maximize its benefits and establish a calming routine.

Benefits of Box Breathing:

• **Stress Reduction**: Box breathing activates the parasympathetic nervous system, which promotes relaxation and reduces the physiological effects of stress. It helps lower heart rate, blood pressure, and cortisol levels.

• **Anxiety Management**: By regulating breathing and promoting a steady rhythm, box breathing can alleviate symptoms of anxiety, including racing thoughts, nervousness, and restlessness.

• **Improved Focus and Concentration**: The structured pattern of box breathing helps enhance mental clarity and concentration. It can be used as a mindfulness practice to improve focus during tasks or before important events.

• **Enhanced Emotional Regulation**: Box breathing encourages controlled breathing and mindfulness, which can improve emotional stability and resilience. It helps individuals manage emotional responses more effectively.

• **Better Sleep Quality**: Practicing box breathing before bedtime can promote relaxation and prepare the body for sleep. It can help reduce insomnia symptoms and improve overall sleep quality.

• **Cognitive Benefits**: Box breathing supports cognitive function by increasing oxygenation and circulation to the brain. This can enhance alertness, memory retention, and overall cognitive performance.

• **Physical Benefits**: Regular practice of box breathing can improve respiratory efficiency, increase lung capacity, and optimize oxygen uptake. It supports overall respiratory health and endurance.

Tips for Practicing Box Breathing:

- **Start Slowly**: Begin with shorter sessions of box breathing (e.g., 1-2 minutes) and gradually increase the duration as you become more comfortable with the technique.

- **Consistency**: Incorporate box breathing into your daily routine or use it as needed during stressful situations to maintain its effectiveness.

- **Combine with Mindfulness**: Focus on the sensations of your breath during box breathing to enhance mindfulness and deepen relaxation.

- **Adjust Counts**: Modify the duration of each count (inhalation, holding, exhalation, holding) to suit your comfort level and respiratory capacity.

Box breathing is a versatile and accessible technique that can be practiced anywhere and at any time to promote relaxation, reduce stress, and enhance overall well-being.

Integrating this simple yet effective breathing exercise into your daily life can provide numerous mental, emotional, and physical benefits.

Yoga Poses And Sequences That Stimulate The Vagus Nerve

Yoga can be a powerful tool for stimulating the vagus nerve, which plays a crucial role in regulating the parasympathetic nervous system and promoting relaxation and stress reduction. Here are some yoga poses and sequences that are known to stimulate the vagus nerve:

Yoga Poses:

Deep Breathing (Pranayama):

- **Technique**: Focus on deep diaphragmatic breathing (abdominal breathing) or alternate nostril breathing (Nadi Shodhana Pranayama) to enhance vagal tone and activate the parasympathetic nervous system.

Child's Pose (Balasana):

- **Technique**: Kneel on the mat, sit back on your heels, and stretch your arms forward with your forehead resting on the mat. This gentle forward fold and compression of the abdomen can stimulate the vagus nerve.

Fish Pose (Matsyasana):

- **Technique**: Lie on your back with your legs extended and feet together. Place your hands palms-down under your buttocks. Inhale, press your forearms and elbows into the floor, lift your chest, and tilt your head back. This pose can stretch the neck and throat, potentially stimulating the vagus nerve.

Bridge Pose (Setu Bandhasana):

- **Technique**: Lie on your back with your knees bent and feet hip-width apart. Press your feet and arms into the mat as you lift your hips towards the ceiling. This backbend opens the chest and stimulates the vagus nerve.

Cat-Cow Pose (Marjaryasana-Bitilasana):

• **Technique**: Start on your hands and knees, with your wrists aligned under your shoulders and knees under your hips. Inhale as you arch your back, lifting your tailbone and chest (Cow Pose). Exhale as you round your spine, tucking your chin towards your chest (Cat Pose). This gentle flow can stimulate the vagus nerve through spinal movement and breath coordination.

Corpse Pose (Savasana):

• **Technique**: Lie flat on your back with your arms and legs extended, palms facing up. Close your eyes and relax your entire body. Focus on deep, slow breathing and allow your mind to become quiet. Savasana promotes relaxation and can help activate the parasympathetic nervous system.

Yoga Sequences:

Vinyasa Flow with Breath Emphasis:

• **Sequence**: Start with gentle warm-up poses such as Cat-Cow, Child's Pose, and gentle twists. Move into a sequence of standing poses like Warrior poses (Virabhadrasana series), Triangle Pose (Trikonasana), and Tree Pose (Vrksasana). End with cooling-down poses such as Bridge Pose and Savasana, focusing on deep breathing throughout.

Restorative Yoga Sequence:

• **Sequence**: Include supportive poses like Supported Bridge Pose (using a block under the sacrum), Supported Child's Pose (using a bolster), and Reclining Bound Angle Pose (Supta Baddha Konasana). Hold each pose for several minutes, focusing on deep, relaxed breathing and allowing the body to release tension.

Yin Yoga Sequence:

- **Sequence**: Practice long-held poses such as Sphinx Pose, Thread the Needle Pose (Parsva Balasana), and Butterfly Pose (Baddha Konasana). These poses target the spine and hips, facilitating relaxation and potentially stimulating the vagus nerve.

Tips for Practicing:

- **Focus on Breath**: Coordinate movement with deep, mindful breathing to enhance the stimulation of the vagus nerve.

- **Mindfulness**: Stay present and aware of sensations in the body during each pose and sequence to deepen the mind-body connection.

- **Comfort and Support**: Use props like blocks, bolsters, and blankets to support your body and ensure comfort in poses, especially in restorative and yin yoga practices.

- **Consistency**: Practice regularly to experience the cumulative benefits of yoga on vagal tone and overall well-being.

Integrating these yoga poses and sequences into your routine can help promote relaxation, reduce stress, and support vagal tone, fostering a sense of calm and balance in both body and mind.

Yoga's Impact On Vagal Tone

Yoga has a profound impact on vagal tone, primarily through its ability to activate the parasympathetic nervous system and stimulate the vagus nerve. Here's how yoga positively influences vagal tone and overall well-being:

Mechanisms of Impact:

Breathing Practices (Pranayama):

- **Deep Breathing**: Practices such as diaphragmatic breathing (abdominal breathing), alternate nostril breathing (Nadi Shodhana), and extended exhalation techniques enhance vagal tone. These techniques involve slow, controlled breathing patterns that stimulate the vagus nerve and promote relaxation.

Mindfulness and Relaxation:

- **Yoga Poses**: Gentle stretching, mindful movement, and holding poses (asanas) improve body awareness and relaxation. Poses like Child's Pose (Balasana), Corpse Pose (Savasana), and forward bends activate the relaxation response, supporting vagal activation.

Physical Benefits:

- **Stretching and Muscle Relaxation**: Yoga poses increase blood flow, stretch muscles, and reduce physical tension. This enhances circulation and promotes relaxation, which positively impacts vagal tone and overall autonomic balance.

Heart Rate Variability (HRV):

• **Vagal Activation**: Yoga practices have been shown to increase heart rate variability (HRV), which reflects the body's ability to adapt to stress and regulate the autonomic nervous system. Higher HRV indicates stronger vagal tone and improved resilience to stress.

Emotional Regulation:

• **Stress Reduction**: Yoga reduces cortisol levels (stress hormone) and activates the parasympathetic nervous system. This helps regulate emotions, reduce anxiety and depression symptoms, and improve overall mood, all of which are influenced by vagal tone.

Specific Yoga Practices for Vagal Tone:

• **Restorative Yoga**: Focuses on gentle poses held for longer durations, promoting deep relaxation and vagal activation.

• **Pranayama Techniques**: Includes breath control practices that directly influence vagal tone, such as slow breathing, extended exhalations, and alternate nostril breathing.

• **Mindfulness Meditation**: Combines focused attention and awareness of breath and body sensations to enhance vagal tone and reduce stress.

• **Yin Yoga**: Involves passive stretching and long holds in poses that target connective tissues, promoting relaxation and improving vagal tone over time.

Benefits of Improved Vagal Tone:

- **Stress Resilience**: Enhanced vagal tone supports better stress management and resilience, reducing the physiological and psychological impacts of chronic stress.

- **Heart Health**: Optimal vagal tone regulates heart rate variability, promoting cardiovascular health and reducing the risk of heart disease.

- **Digestive Health**: Vagal tone influences digestive processes, including stomach acid production and gut motility, supporting better digestion and nutrient absorption.

- **Emotional Well-being**: Improved vagal tone correlates with better emotional regulation, reduced anxiety, and enhanced overall well-being.

Integration into Daily Life:

- **Consistency**: Regular practice of yoga, including breathwork and relaxation techniques, maximizes the benefits on vagal tone and overall health.

- **Holistic Approach**: Combine yoga with healthy lifestyle choices, such as balanced nutrition, adequate sleep, and regular physical activity, to optimize vagal tone and well-being.

Yoga's impact on vagal tone is profound and multifaceted, promoting relaxation, stress reduction, and overall autonomic balance through its integrated approach to breath, movement, and mindfulness. By incorporating yoga into your routine, you can enhance vagal tone and cultivate greater resilience to stress while fostering holistic well-being.

CHAPTER SIX
Mindfulness Practices And Their Effects On The Vagus Nerve

Mindfulness practices have been shown to positively impact the vagus nerve and enhance vagal tone, primarily through their effects on stress reduction, emotional regulation, and overall well-being. Here's how mindfulness practices influence the vagus nerve:

Understanding Vagal Tone and Mindfulness:

Vagal Tone and the Parasympathetic Nervous System:

• The vagus nerve is a key component of the parasympathetic nervous system (PNS), often referred to as the "rest-and-digest" system. It helps regulate bodily functions at rest, including heart rate, digestion, and immune response. Higher vagal tone is associated with greater resilience to stress and better overall health.

Impact of Mindfulness Practices:

- **Focused Attention**: Mindfulness involves paying attention to the present moment without judgment. Practices such as mindful breathing, body scan meditation, and mindful movement (e.g., yoga) cultivate awareness and strengthen the mind-body connection.

- **Stress Reduction**: Mindfulness practices reduce physiological markers of stress, such as cortisol levels and sympathetic nervous system activation (fight-or-flight response). By promoting relaxation and calming the mind, mindfulness enhances vagal activation and improves vagal tone.

- **Emotional Regulation**: Mindfulness enhances the ability to regulate emotions by increasing prefrontal cortex activity, which influences the vagus nerve and parasympathetic function. This supports adaptive responses to stress and reduces emotional reactivity.

- **Resilience to Stress**: Regular mindfulness practice improves resilience to stressors by enhancing coping mechanisms and reducing the impact of chronic stress on the body. This resilience is partly mediated through improved vagal tone and autonomic nervous system balance.

Mindfulness Practices That Influence Vagal Tone:

Mindful Breathing:

- **Technique**: Focus on slow, deep diaphragmatic breathing. Pay attention to the sensations of the breath entering and leaving the body. This practice activates the vagus nerve and promotes relaxation.

Body Scan Meditation:

- **Technique**: Gradually scan through different parts of the body, observing sensations without judgment. This practice enhances body awareness and relaxes tension, indirectly supporting vagal tone.

Loving-Kindness Meditation (Metta):

- **Technique**: Cultivate feelings of compassion and goodwill towards oneself and others. This practice enhances positive emotions, which are associated with improved vagal tone and emotional well-being.

Yoga and Mindful Movement:

- **Technique**: Engage in yoga poses that emphasize deep breathing and mindful awareness of body movements. Practices like gentle stretching, slow transitions between poses, and mindful attention to alignment promote relaxation and vagal activation.

Mindfulness in Daily Activities:

- **Technique**: Practice mindfulness in everyday tasks such as eating, walking, or listening attentively to others. By staying present and aware, you can reduce stress levels and enhance vagal tone throughout the day.

Benefits of Improved Vagal Tone:

- **Enhanced Relaxation**: Improved vagal tone promotes a sense of calmness and relaxation, reducing the physiological effects of stress on the body.

- **Improved Emotional Well-being**: Strong vagal tone supports emotional resilience, reduces anxiety and depression symptoms, and enhances overall mood stability.

- **Better Physical Health**: Optimal vagal tone is associated with improved cardiovascular function, digestive health, and immune response, contributing to overall well-being.

Integration into Daily Life:

- **Consistency**: Regular practice of mindfulness techniques enhances their effectiveness in improving vagal tone and overall health.

- **Mind-Body Connection**: Cultivate a mindful approach to life, integrating awareness, compassion, and acceptance into daily activities to support vagal activation and emotional balance.

Mindfulness practices play a significant role in improving vagal tone by reducing stress, enhancing emotional regulation, and fostering a deeper mind-body connection. By incorporating mindfulness into your routine, you can promote relaxation, resilience, and overall well-being through enhanced vagal function.

Aerobic Exercises And Their Impact On Vagal Tone

Aerobic exercises, also known as cardio exercises, have a notable impact on vagal tone and overall autonomic nervous system function. Here's how aerobic exercises influence vagal tone and contribute to overall well-being:

Understanding Vagal Tone and Aerobic Exercise:

Vagal Tone and the Autonomic Nervous System:

• The vagus nerve is a key component of the parasympathetic nervous system (PNS), which regulates relaxation responses and counters the sympathetic nervous system's (SNS) stress response (fight-or-flight).

Impact of Aerobic Exercise:

- **Increased Heart Rate Variability (HRV)**: Aerobic exercise has been shown to increase heart rate variability, which is a marker of vagal tone. Higher HRV reflects the ability of the body to adapt to stress and indicates stronger vagal function.

- **Autonomic Balance**: Regular aerobic exercise promotes a shift towards parasympathetic dominance (vagal activation) during recovery periods after exercise. This helps in faster recovery, reduces heart rate, and promotes relaxation.

- **Reduction in Chronic Stress**: Aerobic exercise lowers cortisol levels (stress hormone) and reduces sympathetic nervous system activity, thereby supporting vagal tone improvement and overall stress reduction.

Types of Aerobic Exercises Beneficial for Vagal Tone:

Moderate-Intensity Cardiovascular Activities:

- **Brisk Walking**: Walking at a moderate pace increases heart rate gradually and can be sustained for longer durations, making it beneficial for improving vagal tone.

- **Jogging or Running**: Running and jogging elevate heart rate and promote deeper breathing, enhancing cardiovascular fitness and vagal tone over time.

- **Cycling**: Riding a bicycle at a moderate intensity engages large muscle groups and improves cardiovascular health, contributing to vagal tone enhancement.

- **Swimming**: Swimming provides a full-body workout that improves cardiovascular endurance and promotes relaxation, supporting vagal activation.

High-Intensity Interval Training (HIIT):

- **Interval Training**: Alternating between periods of intense exercise and rest or low-intensity recovery boosts cardiovascular fitness and increases HRV, positively impacting vagal tone.

Benefits of Improved Vagal Tone Through Aerobic Exercise:

- **Stress Reduction**: Enhanced vagal tone helps regulate the body's stress response, leading to reduced anxiety levels and improved emotional resilience.

- **Cardiovascular Health**: Optimal vagal tone supports healthy heart function, regulates blood pressure, and lowers the risk of cardiovascular diseases.

- **Respiratory Efficiency**: Aerobic exercise improves respiratory function and efficiency, enhancing oxygen uptake and supporting overall respiratory health.

- **Improved Mood and Well-being**: Regular aerobic exercise stimulates the release of endorphins (feel-good hormones), promoting a positive mood and overall sense of well-being.

Tips for Incorporating Aerobic Exercise:

- **Consistency**: Aim for at least 150 minutes of moderate-intensity aerobic exercise per week, spread over several days, to maximize the benefits on vagal tone and overall health.

- **Variety**: Incorporate different types of aerobic exercises to keep your routine engaging and to target different muscle groups while promoting cardiovascular fitness.

- **Progression**: Gradually increase the intensity and duration of your workouts as your fitness level improves to continually challenge your cardiovascular system and enhance vagal tone.

- **Recovery**: Allow adequate time for recovery between workouts to optimize adaptation and recovery processes, supporting vagal activation and overall well-being.

Regular participation in aerobic activities contributes to a balanced autonomic nervous system, supporting relaxation, resilience, and optimal physiological function.

CHAPTER SEVEN
Resistance Training And Vagus Nerve Stimulation

Resistance training, also known as strength training or weightlifting, typically involves exercises that challenge the muscles against resistance (such as weights, resistance bands, or body weight).

While aerobic exercise is often emphasized for its cardiovascular benefits, resistance training also plays a role in influencing vagal tone and overall health, albeit through different mechanisms compared to aerobic exercise.

Impact of Resistance Training on Vagal Tone:

Muscle Contraction and Vagal Response:

- Resistance training involves repetitive muscle contractions against resistance. These contractions stimulate mechanoreceptors within the muscles, which in turn send signals to the brain and activate the autonomic nervous system, including the vagus nerve.

Acute Cardiovascular Response:

- During resistance exercises, there is an acute increase in blood pressure and heart rate due to the cardiovascular demands of the workout. This response is followed by a recovery period where the parasympathetic nervous system, including the vagus nerve, helps restore heart rate and blood pressure to resting levels.

Chronic Adaptations and Vagal Tone:

- Over time, regular resistance training can lead to adaptations in the autonomic nervous system. While acute sessions may initially stress the body, chronic training improves overall cardiovascular fitness, enhances heart rate variability (HRV), and supports vagal tone.

Combined Effects with Aerobic Exercise:

- Combining resistance training with aerobic exercise can synergistically improve vagal tone and overall autonomic balance. Both types of exercise provide complementary benefits for cardiovascular health and stress management.

Benefits of Resistance Training on Vagal Tone and Overall Health:

- **Improved Heart Rate Variability (HRV)**: Like aerobic exercise, resistance training can increase HRV, which indicates better vagal tone and enhanced ability to regulate stress responses.

- **Enhanced Cardiovascular Health**: Resistance training improves cardiovascular endurance, muscle strength, and efficiency. This can lower resting heart rate and reduce the workload on the heart, benefiting overall cardiovascular function.

- **Metabolic Health**: Building lean muscle mass through resistance training improves insulin sensitivity and glucose metabolism, supporting metabolic health and reducing the risk of metabolic disorders.

- **Bone Health**: Weight-bearing resistance exercises stimulate bone remodeling and strengthen bones, reducing the risk of osteoporosis and enhancing overall skeletal health.

Tips for Incorporating Resistance Training:

- **Consultation**: Consult with a fitness professional or trainer to develop a personalized resistance training program tailored to your fitness level, goals, and any medical considerations.

- **Progression**: Start with lighter weights or resistance and gradually increase intensity and resistance over time as your strength improves.

- **Variety**: Include a variety of exercises that target different muscle groups, using free weights, machines, resistance bands, or body weight exercises to keep workouts engaging and effective.

- **Rest and Recovery**: Allow adequate time for muscles to recover between resistance training sessions to optimize adaptation and reduce the risk of overtraining.

- **Integration with Aerobic Exercise**: Combine resistance training with aerobic activities for a balanced fitness routine that supports overall health, including cardiovascular and vagal tone benefits.

While resistance training is primarily associated with muscular strength and endurance, it also contributes to improving vagal tone and autonomic nervous system function. Incorporating resistance exercises into your fitness regimen can provide comprehensive health benefits, supporting cardiovascular health, stress management, and overall well-being.

Nutrients And Foods That Support Vagus Nerve Function

Supporting vagus nerve function through nutrition involves consuming foods and nutrients that promote overall nerve health, reduce inflammation, and support the production of neurotransmitters crucial for vagal tone. Here are some nutrients and foods that can help support vagus nerve function:

1. Omega-3 Fatty Acids:

Omega-3 fatty acids are essential for brain health and nerve function. They support the integrity of cell membranes, reduce inflammation, and promote neurotransmitter function. Sources include:

• **Fatty Fish**: Salmon, mackerel, sardines, and trout are rich sources of EPA and DHA, two important types of omega-3 fatty acids.

• **Flaxseeds and Chia Seeds**: These seeds are high in ALA (alpha-linolenic acid), a plant-based omega-3 fatty acid that can be converted to EPA and DHA in the body.

• **Walnuts**: Walnuts are a good source of ALA and also provide antioxidants and other nutrients beneficial for brain health.

2. Antioxidants:

• Antioxidants protect nerve cells from oxidative stress and inflammation, which can damage nerve tissue and affect neurotransmitter function. Foods rich in antioxidants include:

• **Berries**: Blueberries, strawberries, raspberries, and blackberries are rich in antioxidants like flavonoids, which have neuroprotective effects.

• **Dark Chocolate**: Dark chocolate (at least 70% cocoa) contains flavonoids that support brain health and improve blood flow.

• **Green Leafy Vegetables**: Spinach, kale, and Swiss chard are high in antioxidants such as vitamins C and E, which support nerve function.

3. B Vitamins:

B vitamins play a crucial role in nerve health and neurotransmitter synthesis. They help convert food into energy and support the production of myelin, a protective sheath around nerves. Sources include:

- **Whole Grains**: Brown rice, oats, quinoa, and whole wheat provide B vitamins, particularly thiamine (B1), riboflavin (B2), niacin (B3), and folate (B9).

- **Legumes**: Beans, lentils, and chickpeas are rich in B vitamins, especially folate and B6.

- **Leafy Greens**: Spinach, kale, and broccoli contain folate and other B vitamins important for nerve health.

4. Magnesium:

Magnesium plays a role in nerve function and relaxation by regulating neurotransmitters and neuromuscular function. Good sources include:

- **Nuts and Seeds**: Almonds, cashews, and pumpkin seeds are rich in magnesium.

- **Whole Grains**: Whole wheat, brown rice, and oats provide magnesium along with B vitamins.

- **Dark Leafy Greens**: Spinach, Swiss chard, and kale are good sources of magnesium.

5. Probiotics:

A healthy gut microbiome supports overall health, including brain function and neurotransmitter production. Probiotic-rich foods include:

- **Yogurt**: Choose plain, unsweetened yogurt with live cultures for probiotic benefits.

- **Kefir**: A fermented dairy product that provides probiotics and beneficial bacteria.

- **Kimchi and Sauerkraut**: Fermented vegetables that support gut health and provide probiotics.

6. Polyphenols:

Polyphenols are plant compounds with antioxidant and anti-inflammatory properties that support brain health and nerve function. Sources include:

- **Green Tea**: Contains catechins, a type of polyphenol with neuroprotective effects.

- **Turmeric**: Contains curcumin, a potent anti-inflammatory compound that supports brain health.

- **Red Wine**: In moderation, red wine contains resveratrol, a polyphenol that supports heart health and may benefit nerve function.

Tips for Supporting Vagus Nerve Function:

- **Balanced Diet**: Eat a balanced diet rich in whole foods, including fruits, vegetables, lean proteins, and healthy fats, to support overall nerve health.

- **Hydration**: Drink plenty of water throughout the day to support nerve function and overall health.

- **Avoid Inflammatory Foods**: Limit processed foods, refined sugars, and excessive alcohol consumption, which can contribute to inflammation and affect nerve health.

- **Mindful Eating**: Practice mindful eating habits to support digestion and nutrient absorption, which indirectly supports vagus nerve function.

Incorporating these nutrient-rich foods into your diet can support vagus nerve function, promote overall nerve health, and contribute to overall well-being and cognitive function.

CHAPTER EIGHT
Cold Exposure And Vagal Response

Cold exposure can stimulate the vagus nerve and elicit a variety of physiological responses that contribute to overall health and well-being. Here's how cold exposure impacts vagal response and its potential benefits:

Mechanisms of Cold Exposure and Vagal Response:

Vasoconstriction and Vagal Activation:

- Cold exposure causes vasoconstriction, which is the narrowing of blood vessels to conserve heat. This triggers a reflex response involving the vagus nerve, leading to a decrease in heart rate (bradycardia) and blood pressure.

Breathing and Respiratory Changes:

• Exposure to cold can lead to changes in breathing patterns, such as deeper inhalations and slower exhalations, which are associated with vagal activation and increased parasympathetic activity.

Brown Adipose Tissue (BAT) Activation:

• Cold exposure stimulates the activation of brown adipose tissue (BAT), a type of fat tissue that generates heat through thermogenesis. BAT activation is mediated by the sympathetic nervous system but also involves vagal pathways to regulate energy balance.

Immune Modulation and Inflammation:

- Cold exposure may modulate immune function and reduce inflammation through vagal pathways. Vagal activation can suppress pro-inflammatory cytokine production and promote anti-inflammatory responses, contributing to immune regulation.

Potential Benefits of Cold Exposure on Vagal Response:

Enhanced Heart Rate Variability (HRV):

- Cold exposure has been shown to increase HRV, indicating improved vagal tone and autonomic balance. Higher HRV is associated with better cardiovascular health, stress resilience, and overall well-being.

Improved Stress Resilience:

- Regular exposure to cold may enhance resilience to stress by strengthening vagal responses and improving the body's ability to adapt to environmental stressors.

Mood Regulation:

- Cold exposure has been linked to mood improvement and mental clarity, possibly through vagal modulation and the release of endorphins and neurotransmitters associated with well-being.

Metabolic Benefits:

- Cold exposure, particularly through techniques like cold showers or cold water immersion (cryotherapy), can promote metabolic health by increasing energy expenditure, enhancing insulin sensitivity, and supporting weight management.

Types of Cold Exposure:

- **Cold Water Immersion**: Briefly immersing the body in cold water, such as cold showers or ice baths, stimulates rapid vasoconstriction and activates the sympathetic nervous system, followed by a parasympathetic rebound.

- **Cold Air Exposure**: Spending time in cold environments, such as outdoor activities in colder climates or exposure to cold air, can elicit similar physiological responses and stimulate vagal pathways.

Safety Considerations:

- **Gradual Adaptation**: Start with shorter exposures to cold and gradually increase duration and intensity to allow the body to adapt safely.

- **Individual Variability**: Responses to cold exposure can vary among individuals based on age, health status, and tolerance levels. Consult with a healthcare professional before beginning any new cold exposure regimen, especially if you have pre-existing health conditions.

- **Hydration and Warm-Up**: Stay hydrated and warm up properly before and after cold exposure to support cardiovascular function and prevent hypothermia or other adverse effects.

Cold exposure can positively impact vagal response through mechanisms such as vasoconstriction, respiratory changes, and immune modulation. Incorporating controlled cold exposure techniques into your routine may enhance vagal tone, improve stress resilience, and support overall health and well-being.

Massage Therapy And Its Effects On The Vagus Nerve

Massage therapy can have beneficial effects on the vagus nerve and the autonomic nervous system, contributing to relaxation, stress reduction, and overall well-being. Here's how massage therapy influences the vagus nerve and its potential effects:

Mechanisms of Massage Therapy and Vagal Stimulation:

Relaxation Response:

- Massage therapy promotes relaxation by reducing muscle tension, lowering heart rate, and enhancing blood circulation. These physiological changes are associated with increased parasympathetic activity, including vagal tone.

Mechanical Pressure and Nerve Stimulation:

- Gentle pressure applied during massage can stimulate mechanoreceptors in the skin, muscles, and connective tissues. This stimulation sends signals to the brain, activating the parasympathetic nervous system, including the vagus nerve.

Reduction in Stress Hormones:

- Massage therapy has been shown to decrease levels of stress hormones such as cortisol and increase levels of serotonin and dopamine, neurotransmitters associated with relaxation and mood improvement. These neurochemical changes are mediated in part by vagal pathways.

Enhanced Heart Rate Variability (HRV):

- Studies have indicated that massage therapy can improve heart rate variability (HRV), a marker of vagal tone and autonomic balance. Higher HRV reflects greater adaptability to stress and better overall cardiovascular health.

Potential Effects of Massage Therapy on Vagal Tone:

- **Improved Stress Resilience**: Regular massage sessions can help regulate the body's stress response, reduce chronic stress levels, and improve the body's ability to recover from stressors, supported by enhanced vagal activation.

- **Emotional Well-being**: Massage therapy promotes feelings of relaxation, calmness, and emotional balance, which are influenced by vagal tone and parasympathetic activity.

- **Digestive Health**: Vagus nerve stimulation through massage may improve digestion and gut motility, as the vagus nerve plays a crucial role in regulating gastrointestinal functions.

- **Pain Management**: Massage therapy can alleviate muscular tension and reduce pain perception, possibly through vagal modulation and the release of endorphins and other pain-relieving neurotransmitters.

Types of Massage Therapy Beneficial for Vagal Activation:

- **Swedish Massage**: This gentle, relaxing massage technique involves long strokes, kneading, and circular movements to promote relaxation and vagal activation.

- **Deep Tissue Massage**: Focuses on deeper layers of muscle tissue to release chronic tension and improve circulation, potentially stimulating vagal responses.

- **Aromatherapy Massage**: Combines massage with essential oils known for their relaxation and stress-relief properties, enhancing the overall therapeutic benefits on vagal tone.

- **Craniosacral Therapy**: A gentle, non-invasive technique that targets the craniosacral system to improve the flow of cerebrospinal fluid and promote relaxation, potentially influencing vagal activity.

Integration into Wellness Practices:

- **Consistency**: Regular sessions of massage therapy can maximize the cumulative benefits on vagal tone and overall health.

- **Holistic Approach**: Combine massage therapy with other stress-reducing practices such as yoga, meditation, and deep breathing exercises to synergistically support vagal activation and emotional well-being.

- **Individualized Approach**: Work with a qualified massage therapist who can tailor the treatment to your specific needs and health goals, ensuring safety and effectiveness.

Massage therapy promotes relaxation, reduces stress, and enhances vagal tone through its effects on the autonomic nervous system. By incorporating massage into your wellness routine, you can support overall health, emotional balance, and resilience to stress, benefiting from improved vagal function and enhanced well-being.

CHAPTER NINE
Creating A Daily Routine

Creating a daily routine can significantly enhance productivity, well-being, and overall satisfaction with life. Here's a structured approach to creating an effective daily routine:

1. Identify Your Goals and Priorities:

- **Reflect on what matters**: Consider your short-term and long-term goals, as well as your values and priorities in life.

- **Set specific objectives**: Determine what you want to achieve daily, whether it's related to work, health, personal development, relationships, or other aspects of your life.

2. Time Blocking and Scheduling:

- **Allocate time for activities**: Divide your day into blocks of time dedicated to specific tasks or types of activities (e.g., work, exercise, leisure, family time).

• **Prioritize tasks**: Schedule your most important and challenging tasks during your peak energy hours when you are most focused and productive.

• **Include buffer time**: Allow for breaks between tasks to rest, recharge, and transition smoothly.

3. Morning Routine:

• **Start your day intentionally**: Incorporate activities that set a positive tone for the day, such as mindfulness, exercise, journaling, or a healthy breakfast.

• **Review your goals**: Take a few minutes to review your goals and prioritize your tasks for the day.

4. Work or Productive Time:

- **Focus on deep work**: Dedicate uninterrupted blocks of time to tasks that require concentration and creativity.

- **Manage distractions**: Minimize interruptions by turning off notifications, setting boundaries, and creating a conducive work environment.

5. Breaks and Physical Activity:

- **Take regular breaks**: Schedule short breaks throughout the day to stretch, walk, or do breathing exercises to refresh your mind and body.

- **Incorporate exercise**: Include physical activity, whether it's a workout, yoga session, or a walk outdoors, to boost energy levels and promote overall health.

6. Meal Times and Nutrition:

- **Plan healthy meals**: Prepare nutritious meals and snacks ahead of time to maintain energy levels and support overall well-being.

- **Mindful eating**: Take time to enjoy your meals without distractions, focusing on nourishing your body and mind.

7. Evening Routine:

- **Wind down**: Include activities that signal the end of the day and promote relaxation, such as reading, meditating, or practicing gratitude.

- **Review your day**: Reflect on your accomplishments, challenges, and lessons learned. Plan for the next day by prioritizing tasks.

8. Self-Care and Personal Development:

- **Schedule time for self-care**: Incorporate activities that promote mental and emotional well-being, such as hobbies, self-reflection, or spending time with loved ones.

- **Continuous learning**: Set aside time for personal development, whether it's reading books, taking courses, or learning new skills.

9. Consistency and Flexibility:

- **Establish a routine**: Stick to your schedule consistently to build habits and maintain momentum towards your goals.

- **Be flexible**: Allow for adjustments as needed to accommodate unexpected events or changes in priorities without feeling stressed or overwhelmed.

10. Monitor and Adjust:

- **Track your progress**: Keep a journal or use apps to track your daily activities, accomplishments, and areas for improvement.

- **Reflect and adjust**: Regularly review your routine to assess what's working well and where adjustments are needed to optimize your productivity and well-being.

Improve your productivity, improve your overall health and well-being, and cultivate a sense of fulfillment in your daily life by establishing a balanced daily routine that is in accordance with your goals and priorities.

Conclusion

A potent instrument for improving productivity, well-being, and overall life satisfaction is the establishment of a structured daily routine. You can optimize your day to achieve both short-term tasks and long-term aspirations by identifying your objectives, prioritizing tasks, and allocating time effectively.

A balanced approach to daily life is cultivated by incorporating elements such as morning rituals for intention setting, focused work periods, regular pauses for rejuvenation, and mindful activities for self-care.

Furthermore, the integration of healthy behaviors, such as regular physical activity, nutritious eating, and dedicated time for personal growth and relaxation, not only promotes physical health but also improves emotional resilience and mental clarity.

Maintaining a consistent routine while remaining adaptable to unforeseen changes promotes stress reduction and adaptability. In the final analysis, a well-designed daily routine serves as a foundation for success, allowing you to effectively confront daily obstacles, maintain motivation, and develop a life that is both purposeful and fulfilling.

You can maintain productivity, promote well-being, and encourage ongoing development in all facets of your life by consistently assessing and improving your routine in response to personal reflection and feedback.

THE END

www.ingramcontent.com/pod-product-compliance
Lightning Source LLC
Chambersburg PA
CBHW071834210526
45479CB00001B/127